Eyes Wide Open: Understanding Macular Degeneration

Rodney Reynolds

Published by Rodney Reynolds, 2024.

EYES WIDE OPEN: UNDERSTANDING MACULAR DEGENERATION

First edition. January 26, 2024.

Copyright © 2024 Rodney Reynolds.

ISBN: 979-8224990078

Written by Rodney Reynolds.

Table of Contents

Chapter 1: Introduction - Opening Our Eyes to Macular Degeneration

Welcome, dear reader, to a journey that is both enlightening and compassionate – a journey that opens our eyes to the complex world of eyeglasses. These pages explore what we understand and live with and the challenges of this common but often misunderstood eye condition.

The Marvelous Complexity of Sight

Our eyes, that excellent window to the world, give us the unique gift of sight. At the core of this gift is the macula, a small but complex part of the retina that offers our central vision clarity and sharpness. Imagine yourself as a conductor planning a visual ensemble. In this chapter, we unpack the complexities of the eye and explore the delicate dance that allows us to see the beauty around us.

Think of the macula as the eye's ultra-fine camera, capturing every detail, every color, and every detail. That's why you can read a favorite book, admire a piece of art, or see a friend smile. Understanding macular degeneration, a condition that affects this essential part of our vision is critical to understanding how it can profoundly impact how we experience the world.

Embarking on the Macular Journey

Macular degeneration is not just a medical term; It represents a series of progressive eye diseases that affect the macula—dry A.M.D. In the upcoming sections, we will examine the various manifestations of macular degeneration, unpack the complexity of this condition, and highlight its prevalence and potential consequences.

Let's think of a journey with macular degeneration as exploring uncharted territory. It's like embarking on a road trip where the terrain is unknown and landmarks are constantly changing. But don't be afraid; This guide will give us the knowledge and insight to navigate this journey confidently and flexibly.

Through the Lens of Signs and Symptoms

As we move through this review, it is important to recognize the early signs and symptoms that may indicate the presence of cataracts. This chapter is intended as a friendly guide to subtle signs that may need close attention. Distorted central vision, difficulties with facial recognition, or reading difficulties are not just problems but signs that we need to seek treatment promptly.

Consider a set of telescopes in this chapter that will help you capture details you may not see as much. Early detection is like having a map of our journey with myopia – guiding us in the right direction, ensuring we can work in time, and seeking out available treatment options.

Stories That Illuminate

Here in these pages, you will find more than just information; you will meet face-to-face with the lived experiences of individuals facing the challenges of vision loss. Their stories woven into the panel of this chapter add a human touch, allowing them to relate to the situation's complexities.

Meet Sarah, a passionate artist who discovered her passion for painting even after being diagnosed with cataracts. Join James as an avid reader as he shares how audiobooks have become his new window into the world of books. These stories go beyond statistical and medical jargon; they demonstrate the resilience of the human spirit, showing that living with a mirror is not just a limitation but a new way to thrive.

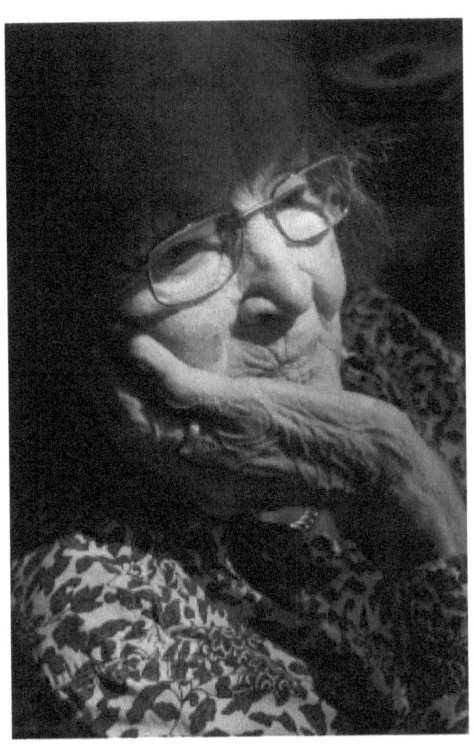

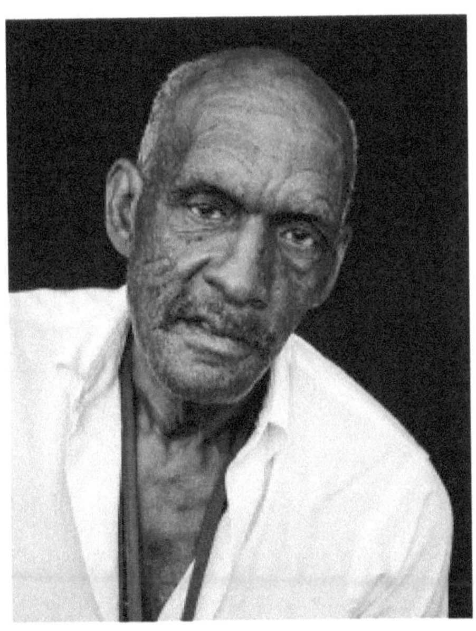

Our Shared Journey Begins

We begin this shared journey with open hearts and friendly tones. Whether you're getting into the twists and turns of eyeglasses yourself, offering support to a loved one, or simply wanting to see your knowledge deepen, this chapter is a warm invitation to explore the world of insight and sympathy.

We also recognize the importance of community support in this journey. This chapter is an actual handshake, welcoming you into the network of individuals who understand, empathize, and share their wisdom. This is a community where questions are encouraged, experiences are celebrated, and no one goes alone.

As we turn the pages together, we celebrate the resilience of the human spirit and find hope that sprouts eternally, even amid visual challenges. This chapter is just the opening act, setting the stage for a story that brings compassion, understanding, and a collective commitment to embracing the beauty of life, which is still alive even through the lenses of rotting glass.

Chapter 2: The Anatomy of Sight: Understanding the Macula

Welcome to the enchanting realm of vision, where the intricate symphony of sight plays out on the grand stage of our eyes. Within the pages of this chapter, we undertake a comprehensive journey delving into the complex anatomy of our eyes, directing our attention toward the diminutive yet awe-inspiring conductor of the visual symphony – the macula.

Cross Section of Eye

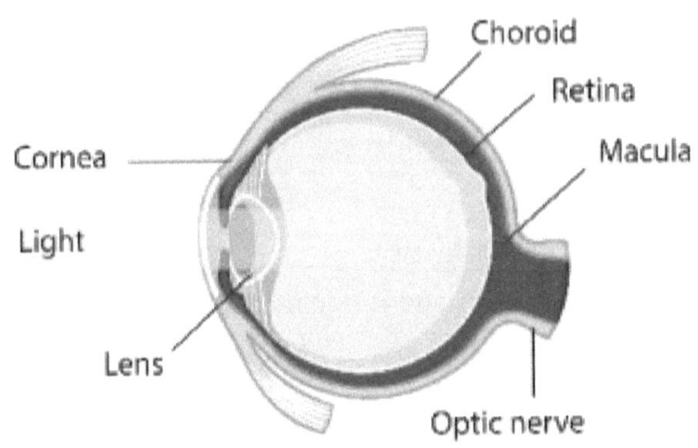

The Maestro of Vision

Picture your eyes as a grand orchestra, harmonizing light, color, and detail into the masterpiece of your visual experience. At the helm is the macula, a diminutive powerhouse nestled within the retina. This unassuming region takes center stage in orchestrating the brilliance of our central vision, akin to the conductor guiding every nuanced note in a musical performance.

Let's begin our exploration with a deeper dive into the eye's cast of characters. The cornea and lens, acting as the natural lenses, meticulously focus light onto the retina—the light-sensitive canvas at the back of the eye. Here, photoreceptor cells, known as rods and cones, capture and process visual information. Enter the macula, the unsung hero responsible for refining this information into the high-definition clarity that defines our ability to read, recognize faces, and appreciate the intricacies of the world.

Unveiling the Macula: A Symphony of Layers

Demystifying the macula reveals a layered masterpiece, each stratum contributing to the symphony of sight. At the core lies the fovea, the crown jewel of the macula, densely packed with cones—photoreceptor cells specializing in color perception and detailed vision. As we peel back the layers, the inner nuclear layer houses the cell bodies of these photoreceptors. In contrast, the outer nuclear layer houses the supporting cells crucial for their sustenance. The retinal pigment epithelium, a protective shield, plays a vital role in nourishing and recycling these delicate cells.

Delving deeper into the intricacies of the macula, we encounter Müller cells, which span from the inner to the outer layers, providing structural support and actively contributing to the overall well-being of this extraordinary region. These cells are akin to architects, ensuring the stability of the macular structure and promoting seamless visual information.

Dancing with Photoreceptors: A Ballet of Precision

The dance of photoreceptor cells within the macula is a ballet of extraordinary precision. Cones, exquisite in their sensitivity to bright light and masters of color vision, gather in abundance within this small but potent region. Proficient in low-light conditions and peripheral vision, Rods waltzs gracefully in the periphery. Together, they choreograph a dynamic visual spectacle, allowing us to revel in the vivid tapestry of our surroundings.

But this dance has its challenges. The balance between the number of cones and rods, the optimal distribution of these cells, and the intricate interplay of neurotransmitters—all contribute to the delicate choreography that enables our eyes to perceive the world with astonishing clarity.

As we plunge into the intricacies of the macula, its significance as the epicenter of visual function becomes increasingly apparent. This small, unassuming region is a powerhouse, seamlessly capturing, processing, and transmitting visual information. This intricate dance lays the foundation for appreciating the profound impact that macular degeneration can exert on our vision.

Guardians of Vision: Blood Supply and Beyond

Akin to any vital organ, the macula relies on a robust blood supply for sustenance. The choroid, a layer beneath the retina, emerges as a guardian, delivering essential nutrients and oxygen to the macula. Understanding this delicate balance elucidates why disruptions, as observed in certain forms of macular degeneration, can profoundly influence vision.

The macula isn't merely a physical entity within our eyes; it emerges as a nexus of vision, a sacred space where the alchemy of sight unfolds. As we progress on this journey, let's carry forward this newfound appreciation for the macula, recognizing it as the linchpin of our visual symphony. Join us as we continue our expedition, delving even deeper into the intricacies of this remarkable structure and unraveling the profound impact its health holds over the orchestration of our sight.

Chapter 3: Seeing the Signs: Early Detection and Diagnosis

Welcome to a pivotal chapter in our exploration of eye health. Here, we navigate the critical terrain of early detection and diagnosis, shedding light on the subtle signals our eyes send us and the essential role timely awareness plays in preserving our vision.

The Silent Language of the Eyes

Our eyes possess a silent language, a nuanced communication that conveys more than meets the eye. In this section, we embark on an in-depth journey into the signs that might serve as early whispers of changes occurring within our visual realm. Consider it a friendly guide, equipping you with the knowledge to decipher this silent language and helping you become attuned to the messages your eyes may be sending.

- Visual Distortions: Deciphering the Ripples

Visual distortions often manifest as subtle ripples in the clarity of our sight. It might be a wavering line in a book or a distortion in the edges of objects. These seemingly innocuous signs can be early indicators of changes in the macula, prompting us to pay closer attention to the intricate dance of our vision.

Let's take a moment to imagine reading a beloved book – a task that usually brings joy. If you find that the lines blur or distort, like a river losing its course, it's a call to action. Consider it your eyes' way of inviting you to explore further, to understand the source of these visual ripples.

- A Palette of Colors: Unraveling Hue Changes

Hues are lively threads that intricately weave the fabric of our visual encounter. When these hues shift or fade, it can be a sign that something is amiss. Picture a world where the reds lose their warmth, and the blues lose their cool – it's a palette that hints at potential changes in the health of our eyes.

So, if you notice a subtle alteration in how colors present themselves, don't dismiss it as a trick of the light. It could be your eyes gently nudging you to seek a deeper understanding of what lies beneath the surface. 3. Central Vision Challenges: Navigating the Maze

Our central vision is like the compass guiding us through the intricacies of daily life. When this compass begins to falter, it's time to take notice. Reading, recognizing faces, or driving may become more challenging. The maze of daily activities might suddenly seem a bit more perplexing.

Imagine threading a needle, and the eye struggles to focus on the fine details. This could be a clue that your central vision, orchestrated by the macula, is changing. Acknowledging these challenges is the first step in navigating the maze and seeking assistance.

- Gradual Blurring: Recognizing the Haze

Blurring, like a gentle fog settling over our vision, is another sign that warrants attention. It might start gradually, imperceptibly altering the sharpness of the world around us. Tasks that were once effortlessly clear may begin to lose their focus.

Think of it as a camera lens slowly drifting out of focus – a phenomenon that beckons us to consider the health of our eyes and explore the possibility of early intervention.

The Journey to Diagnosis

Recognizing these early signs is akin to deciphering a code, and the next step in our journey is understanding how these clues lead us to a formal diagnosis. Friendly reminder: this journey is not a solo expedition but a collaborative effort between you, your eye care professional, and the wealth of medical expertise available.

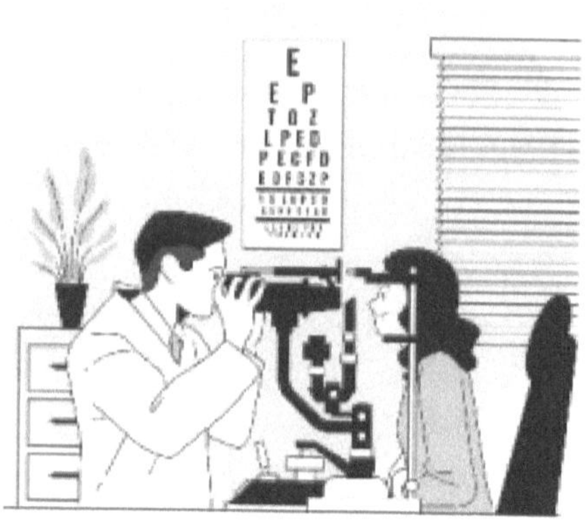

- Comprehensive Eye Exams: Peering into the Depths

Comprehensive eye exams are the cornerstone of early diagnosis.

Comprehensive eye exams encompass a detailed evaluation of your visual acuity, intraocular pressure, and the overall health of your eyes. Your eye care professional may employ advanced imaging techniques or conduct a dilated eye exam, peering into the depths of your eyes to evaluate the condition of the retina, including the macula.

Think of it as a detective unraveling a mystery. The eye care professional, armed with specialized tools and knowledge, navigates the intricate details of your eyes, uncovering clues that might not be visible to the naked eye.

A Dialogue of Symptoms: Sharing Your Story

Your experience is a crucial piece of the puzzle. Engage in a dialogue with your eye care professional, sharing the subtleties of what you've observed. The visual distortions, color shifts, or central vision challenges are part of your unique narrative, and this dialogue helps shape the direction of the investigation.

Consider this conversation a collaborative e ort, where your insights guide the examination and contribute valuable information to the diagnostic process.

- Advanced Imaging and Technology: A Closer Look

Technological advancements offer a more detailed look at the eye's inner workings. Optical coherence tomography (OCT) and fundus photography allow your eye care professional to capture high-resolution images of the retina, providing a roadmap to the intricate landscape of your eyes.

Imagine using a magnifying glass to explore the details of a painting. These technologies enable a deeper understanding of the structural changes within the eye, aiding in early detection and precise diagnosis.

- Monitoring Progress: A Continuous Journey

Early detection is not a one-time event but a continuous journey. Even if you haven't noticed significant changes, regular eye check-ups play a pivotal role in monitoring the health of your eyes. They offer an opportunity to catch subtle shifts before they become more pronounced, allowing for timely intervention and management.

Think of it as tuning an instrument regularly to ensure it produces the most harmonious notes. Regular eye check-ups help maintain the symphony of your vision, ensuring it remains in tune and vibrant.

Facing the Unknown with Knowledge

Embarking on the early detection and diagnosis journey may seem daunting, but knowledge is a powerful ally. Remember, these signs are not roadblocks but guideposts, gently nudging us to pay attention to the intricate language of our eyes.

Consider this chapter as your trusted companion for preserving your vision. By recognizing the signs, engaging in open dialogues with your eye care professional, and embracing the advancements in diagnostic technologies, you empower yourself in the face of the unknown.

In the chapters, we'll explore the avenues of treatment, resilience, and the shared experiences of those who have navigated similar journeys.

Together, we step into the future armed with knowledge, compassion, and the determination to face the unknown with clarity and courage.

Chapter 4: Through the Patient's Lens: Personal Stories of Macular Degeneration

Welcome to a chapter woven with the threads of resilience, courage, and the indomitable spirit of those who have traversed the intricate landscape of macular degeneration. Here, we delve into personal narratives, offering an intimate look through the patient's lens. This perspective illuminates not only the challenges but also the triumphs in the face of visual adversity.

Stories that Resonate

In the mosaic of human experience, personal stories are vibrant pieces that create a tapestry of shared understanding. With its unique challenges, macular degeneration draws individuals from diverse walks of life into a standard narrative. This section opens the door to these stories, hoping they resonate with you, inspire you, and foster a sense of connection.

1.   Sarah's Brush with Colors

Meet Sarah, a passionate artist whose world revolves around the vibrant hues of her palette. Sarah's journey with macular degeneration began as subtle distortions in her artwork. The once precise strokes started to waver, and colors lost their clarity. She said, "It was as if someone dimmed the lights on my canvas."

Sarah's story teaches us that creativity can flourish even in adversity. Sarah rekindled her love for art through adaptive techniques and a newfound appreciation for texture. Her narrative stands as a testament to the enduring strength of the human spirit and the capacity to discover beauty in the most unforeseen corners of life.

1.   James's Literary Odyssey

James, an avid reader with a penchant for literature, found his world gradually fading as macular degeneration overshadowed his reading ability. The words on the page blurred, and the narratives he once devoured with ease became elusive. "It was like losing a dear friend," James reflects.

Yet, from this challenge emerged a literary odyssey. Audiobooks became James's newfound companions, allowing him to traverse the vast landscapes of storytelling. James's journey highlights the adaptability of the human mind and the transformative power of embracing new perspectives.

1. Grace's Vision of Connection

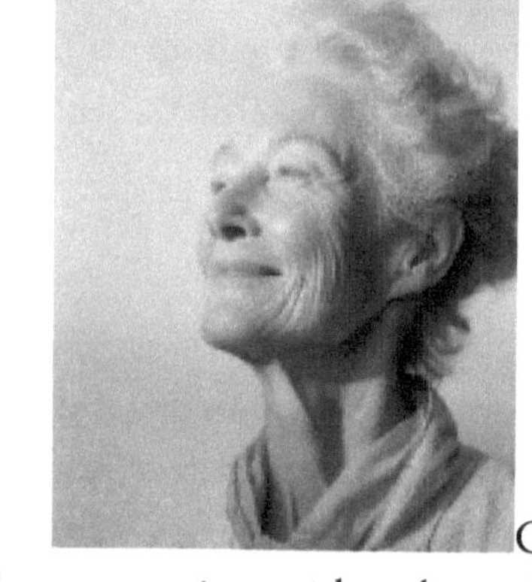

Grace, a social butterfly with a passion for connecting with others, faced the isolating effects of macular degeneration. Recognizing faces in a crowded room became challenging, and the fear of losing connections loomed. "I felt like I was losing a piece of myself," Grace shares.

However, Grace's journey took an unexpected turn. Through support groups and technological aids, she discovered a renewed sense of connection. Her story emphasizes the importance of community and the transformative impact of technology in fostering meaningful relationships.

Common Threads and Shared Wisdom

As we immerse ourselves in these personal narratives, common threads emerge—threads of adaptability, resilience, and the pursuit of joy despite visual challenges. These stories are not just individual accounts but beacons of shared wisdom, offering insights for those navigating similar paths.

1. Adaptation as a Stepping Stone

Sarah, James, and Grace all share a common theme—the ability to adapt. Whether adjusting artistic techniques, embracing audiobooks, or leveraging technology, their stories underscore the importance of flexibility in the face of change. Through adaptation, they preserved their passions and discovered new avenues for self-expression.

1. The Power of Support Systems

Behind each personal story is a support network—family, friends, and fellow individuals facing macular degeneration. These support systems are lifelines, providing emotional sustenance and practical assistance. The experiences of Sarah, James, and Grace illuminate the significance of building and nurturing these connections.

1. Technological Triumphs

Technology emerges as a recurring ally in these narratives. From adaptive tools to innovative devices, the stories showcase the transformative role of technology in enhancing independence and enriching lives. James's embrace of audiobooks and Grace's exploration of assistive technologies illustrate the power of innovation in overcoming visual barriers. Embracing the Journey Ahead

As we navigate these personal stories, we recognize that macular degeneration is not just a medical condition but a shared human experience. Each story, a unique chapter, contributes to a collective narrative of resilience and hope. Through the patient's lens, we better understand the emotional landscape accompanying visual challenges.

The path ahead unfolds like a tapestry, interwoven with strands of resilience, adaptability, and the steadfast essence of the human spirit. In the following chapters, we'll explore practical strategies, innovations, and a deeper understanding of the emotional aspects of living with macular degeneration. Together, we embark on a journey of shared wisdom and empowerment guided by the stories that have shaped the path before us.

Chapter 5: The Science of Shadows: Exploring the Causes of Age-Related Macular Degeneration

The Dance of Genetics and Environment

Welcome to a journey through the intricate landscape of AMD, where we unravel the scientific tapestry that shrouds the causes of this prevalent eye condition. This chapter delves into the underlying factors, exploring the biology, genetics, and environmental influences that cast shadows on the macula.

Imagine our eyes as a delicate dance between our genetic makeup and environment. This dance, while beautifully intricate, also sets the stage for the emergence of AMD. Let's embark on a journey through the science of shadows, understanding the interplay of nature and nurture in shaping the destiny of our vision.

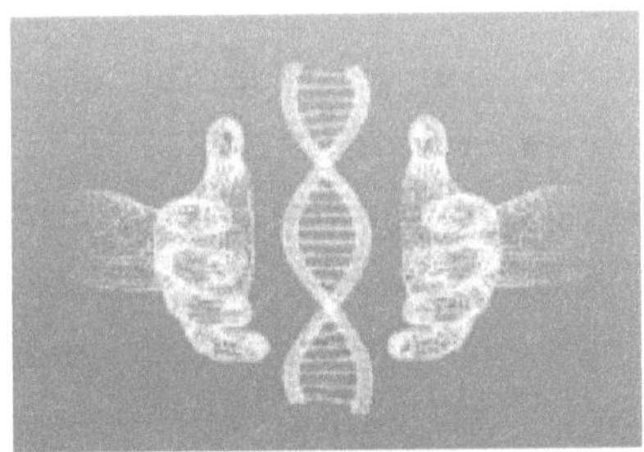

1. Genetics: Unraveling the Genetic Code

The blueprint encoded in our genes significantly influences the likelihood of developing AMD. Picture our genes as a complex code, a script that controls how our eyes age. Specific variations in genes related to the immune system, cholesterol metabolism, and the regulation of blood vessels have been linked to an increased risk of developing AMD.

However, genetics isn't a predetermined fate; it's more like a roadmap with alternative routes. Understanding our genetic predispositions empowers us with knowledge, allowing us to make informed choices and adopt lifestyle measures to mitigate AMD risk.

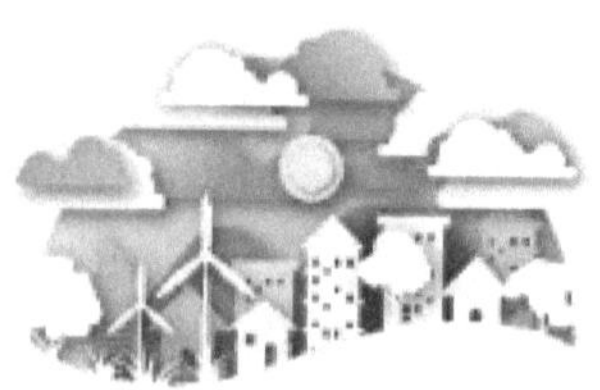

1. Environmental Influences: The Impact of Sunlight and Diet

As we navigate the causes of AMD, the spotlight shifts to our environment. Sunlight has been implicated as a contributing factor with its intricate balance of light and harmful ultraviolet rays. Prolonged exposure to sunlight, especially without adequate protection, may play a role in the development and progression of AMD.

Diet, too, emerges as a key player. Imagine the foods we consume as the fuel that powers the engine of our eyes. Foods rich in antioxidants, like leafy greens, fruits, and fish, offer nourishment that promotes the well-being of our eyes. Conversely, a diet rich in saturated fats and deficient in essential nutrients may contribute to the macula's shadows.

The Intricacies of Inflammation

Inflammation, often dubbed the silent culprit, weaves its thread into the narrative of AMD.

Inflammation, being a natural response to injury or infection, its prolonged or chronic presence can have adverse effects on the delicate structures of the eye, such as the macula.

1. The Immune System's Role: Balancing Act Gone Awry

Our immune system, designed to protect us, can sometimes tip the balance. In AMD, the immune system may mistakenly target healthy cells within the macula, setting off events that ultimately lead to inflammation and subsequent damage. This autoimmune-like response adds another layer of complexity to the science of shadows.

Understanding this intricate dance of the immune system allows us to appreciate the delicate equilibrium required for ocular health. This also creates opportunities for potential therapeutic strategies that seek to regulate the immune response and mitigate the impact of inflammation on the macula.

1. Oxidative Stress: A Culprit in the Shadows

Picture oxidative stress as the aftermath of a storm, where free radicals wreak havoc on the delicate structures of the eye. These unstable molecules, produced as byproducts of normal cellular processes, can accumulate over time, contributing to the aging process of the macula.

Antioxidants, our cellular superheroes, are crucial in neutralizing these free radicals. A deficiency in antioxidants or an imbalance in the body's ability to combat oxidative stress can tip the scales, casting shadows that may lead to the development or progression of AMD.

The Role of Lifestyle and Beyond

Beyond genetics, environment, and inflammation, our lifestyle choices emerge as influential protagonists in the narrative of AMD. Imagine these choices as brushstrokes on the canvas of our health, each one contributing to the overall picture.

1. Smoking: The Cloud of Risk

Smoking, with its tendrils of smoke, casts a dark shadow on eye health. Identified as a notable risk factor for AMD, it hastens the condition's progression. The chemicals in tobacco smoke contribute to oxidative stress, inflammation, and vascular changes—all of which play a role in the development of AMD.

Quitting smoking is akin to lifting the shadows, providing a tangible way to reduce the risk and potentially slow the progression of AMD. It's a transformative choice that opens the door to a brighter, healthier vision.

1. Physical Activity: Illuminating the Path

On the flip side, physical activity emerges as a beacon of light. Regular exercise improves blood circulation, supports overall health, and may protect the macula like a gentle breeze. It's a simple yet powerful lifestyle choice that illuminates the path toward maintaining eye health.

The Ongoing Quest for Understanding

As we conclude this exploration into the causes of AMD, it's essential to recognize that our understanding of this complex condition continues to evolve. Researchers, like explorers in a vast landscape, are uncovering new facets of the science of shadows, leading to innovative treatments and preventive strategies.

This chapter serves as a friendly guide through the scientific intricacies, offering insights that empower you to make informed choices for your eye health. As we journey forward, let's continue illuminating the shadows with knowledge, embracing lifestyle choices that support ocular well-being, and contributing to the quest for a clearer understanding of AMD.

Chapter 6: Navigating Treatment Options: From Medications to Surgery

Welcome to a comprehensive exploration of the diverse avenues for managing macular degeneration. In this chapter, we embark on a journey through the spectrum of treatment options, delving into the intricacies of medications, therapies, and, when necessary, the role of surgery. We aim to provide a nuanced understanding, empowering you to make well-informed decisions customized to your visual needs.

Medications: Targeting the Shadows

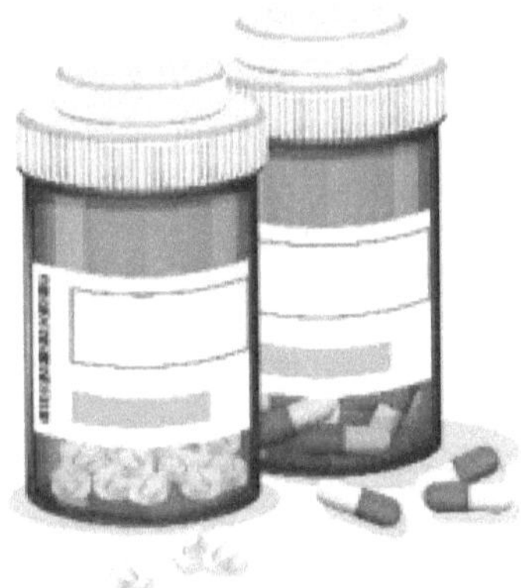

Imagine medications as skilled artists, delicately crafting a canvas of possibilities for managing macular degeneration. From injections to oral medications, these therapeutic options aim to target the underlying causes, slow progression, and, in some cases, restore a semblance of visual clarity.

1. Anti-VEGF Injections: A Precision Strike

Anti-VEGF injections, designed to combat the overproduction of vascular endothelial growth factor (VEGF), a pivotal contributor to the progression of AMD, are the heroes of this narrative. These injections, administered directly into the eye, work like targeted missiles, neutralizing the excessive VEGF and curbing abnormal blood vessel growth.

While eye injections may seem daunting, the procedure is quick and well-tolerated. Many individuals find that the benefits—slowing down disease progression and potentially improving vision—far outweigh any temporary discomfort.

1. Corticosteroids: Taming Inflammation

Corticosteroids step onto the stage as potent inflammation tamers. In some instances, inflammation exacerbates the challenges posed by macular degeneration. Corticosteroid medications, available as injections or implants, suppress inflammation, providing relief and potentially stabilizing the condition.

These treatments highlight the tailored approach to macular degeneration, where the choice of medication depends on each eye's specific characteristics and needs.

Therapies: A Symphony of Support

Beyond medications, envision therapies as the supporting orchestra, enhancing the overall harmony of visual health. These therapies encompass a range of interventions, from laser treatments to photodynamic therapy, each playing a unique role in managing macular degeneration.

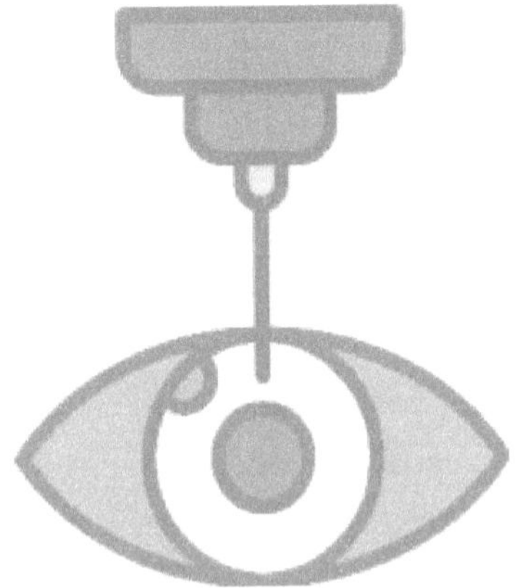

1. Laser Treatments: Precision in Action

Like the conductor's baton, laser treatments guide precise interventions to address abnormal blood vessels. Photocoagulation and photodynamic therapy leverage the power of lasers to seal leaking blood vessels or target specific areas of the macula. These interventions are often employed in specific cases to preserve or improve vision. 2. Low Vision Rehabilitation: A Personalized Symphony

The melody of low vision rehabilitation resonates with individualized support, recognizing that each person's visual needs are unique. Occupational therapists, orientation and mobility specialists, and low-vision optometrists collaborate to enhance daily functioning. This may involve training in adaptive techniques, recommending specialized devices, or providing counseling to navigate the emotional aspects of vision loss.

The Role of Surgery: A Lasting Encore

When the shadows cast by macular degeneration become particularly profound, surgery steps into the spotlight as a lasting encore. While surgical interventions for AMD are relatively uncommon, they are reserved for specific situations where other treatments may not suffice

1. Vitrectomy: Illuminating the Path

Vitrectomy, a surgical procedure entailing the extraction of the vitreous gel in the eye, may be considered in cases of severe vitreous hemorrhage or retinal detachment associated with AMD. This surgery aims to restore or improve vision by clearing the vitreous and addressing complications.

Like any surgical procedure, the decision to undergo vitrectomy is collaborative, involving thorough discussions with your eye care professional to weigh the potential risks and benefits.

The Collaborative Symphony: Your Vision Team

Throughout this journey of treatment options, envision a collaborative symphony where you, as the conductor, lead a team of skilled musicians —your vision care professionals. Whether it's your ophthalmologist, retina specialist, or low-vision therapist, each vision team member plays a crucial role in orchestrating the best possible outcomes.

1. Open Communication: Your Baton of Empowerment

Open communication is your baton of empowerment. Engage in transparent discussions with your vision care professionals about your concerns, goals, and expectations. Your voice guides the symphony, ensuring the treatment options align with your unique needs and preferences.

1. Regular Monitoring: Sustaining the Harmony

Regular monitoring is the sustaining rhythm of this symphony. Scheduled check-ups and follow-ups enable your vision care team to assess the effectiveness of treatments, make adjustments as needed, and ensure the ongoing well-being of your eyes.

Empowering Yourself on the Journey

As you navigate the vast landscape of treatment options for macular degeneration, remember that knowledge is your compass, and empowerment is your guiding star. Each treatment option is a note in the symphony of managing AMD, and together with your vision care team, you can orchestrate a harmonious approach tailored to the nuances of your vision.

In the chapters, we'll delve deeper into lifestyle considerations, emotional well-being, and the ongoing quest for advancements in macular degeneration research. Embrace this chapter as your guide, your companion, as you continue to navigate the journey toward safeguarding and improving the invaluable gift of your vision.

Chapter 7: Living with Low Vision: Practical Strategies for Daily Life

Welcome to a chapter filled with practical insights and friendly guidance on navigating the landscape of low vision. Living with low vision brings unique challenges and opens doors to innovative solutions and adaptive strategies to enhance your daily life. Let's embark on this journey together, exploring practical tips, assistive technologies, and the emotional resilience needed to thrive despite visual challenges.

Understanding Low Vision: A Compassionate Prelude

Living with low vision is akin to exploring a new terrain. In this realm, creativity and adaptability become your trusted companions. This section serves as a compassionate prelude, recognizing the diverse aspects of low vision and laying the foundation for the following practical strategies.

1. Embracing Change: The Heart of Adaptability

At the core of living with low vision is embracing change. Understand that adapting to new ways of doing things is not a sign of limitation but a testament to your resilience. Begin by acknowledging your unique visual needs and cultivating a mindset that welcomes innovation.

1. Building a Support Network: Your Pillars of Strength

Imagine your support network as a fortress, providing strength and assistance when needed. Share your experience with family, friends, and healthcare professionals. Their understanding and support become pillars that help you navigate challenges and celebrate victories, fostering a sense of community.

Practical Tips for Daily Living: Illuminating Your Path

In this section, we delve into the helpful tips illuminating your daily path, making everyday tasks more manageable and enjoyable. These insights cover various aspects of life, from home environment modifications to strategies for reading, writing, and engaging with technology.

1. Optimizing Lighting: Shedding Light on Tasks

Lighting becomes your ally in the world of low vision. Ensure your living spaces are well-lit, with consistent and glare-free illumination. Position task lighting strategically, directing light onto specific areas for enhanced visibility. Experiment with different types of bulbs to find what works best for you.

1. Contrasting Colors: Enhancing Visibility

Contrasting colors provide visual cues that make objects stand out. Choose high-contrast colors for everyday items, such as clothing and kitchen utensils. Using contrasting colors to differentiate between surfaces and objects makes navigating your surroundings easier.

1. Large Print and Bold Fonts: Making Reading Accessible

Transform reading into an accessible and enjoyable activity by opting for large print or bold fonts. Choose books, magazines, and electronic devices that have adjustable text sizes. Experiment with different font styles and background colors to find the combination that maximizes readability.

1. Magnification Tools: Bringing Details Closer

Magnification tools are your visual allies, bringing details closer and enhancing clarity. Explore handheld magnifiers, desktop magnifying lamps, and digital magnification apps. These tools cater to various needs, whether reading fine print or examining intricate details.

1. Audio Books and Text-to-Speech Technology: A Symphony of Voices

Embark on a journey of literature through audiobooks and text-to-speech technology. Let the soothing tones of narrators transport you into captivating stories. Utilize devices and apps that convert written text into spoken words, opening up a world of information and entertainment.

1. Voice-Activated Assistants: Your Virtual Helpers

Welcome virtual helpers into your daily routine. Voice-activated assistants, like smart speakers and virtual assistants on smartphones, respond to your verbal commands, provide information, set reminders, and perform various tasks. These technologies offer hands-free convenience and accessibility.

Enhancing Mobility and Independence: Your Pathway Forward

Navigating the world with low vision involves enhancing mobility and independence. In this section, we explore tips for safe and convenient travel, whether you're walking, using public transportation, or considering guide dogs.

1. White Canes and Mobility Aids: Extending Your Reach

White canes and other mobility aids extend your reach, providing tactile feedback and signaling to others that you have low vision. Familiarize yourself with different cane techniques and consider mobility training to boost your confidence in navigating various environments.

1. Public Transportation Tips: Navigating with Ease

Public transportation can be a reliable means of travel. Familiarize yourself with transportation routes, request assistance if needed, and consider using apps that provide real-time transit information. Public transportation agencies often offer services to accommodate individuals with visual impairments.

1. Guide Dogs: Trusted Companions

Guide dogs are more than assistance animals; they are trusted companions providing guidance and support. If considering a guide dog, connect with reputable guide dog organizations, undergo training, and build a strong bond with your canine partner. Guide dogs enhance mobility and independence while offering companionship.

Embracing Emotional Well-Being: A Vital Harmony

Living with low vision is not just about practical strategies; it's also about nurturing emotional well-being. This section explores the emotional aspects of low vision, offering guidance on building resilience, seeking support, and fostering a positive mindset.

1. Emotional Resilience: Your Inner Strength

Cultivate emotional resilience as your inner strength. Acknowledge the challenges, celebrate your achievements, and recognize the beauty in adaptability. Embrace a growth mindset, viewing challenges as learning and personal growth opportunities.

1. Seeking Support: Connecting with Others

Connect with individuals who share similar experiences. Join support groups, either in person or online, to share insights, exchange practical tips, and build a sense of camaraderie. Peer support can be invaluable in navigating the emotional landscape of low vision.

1. Professional Counseling: A Guiding Light

Professional counseling provides a guiding light for addressing emotional challenges. Consider working with a mental health professional who specializes in low vision or disability-related issues. Counseling offers a safe space to explore emotions, develop coping strategies, and cultivate a positive mindset.

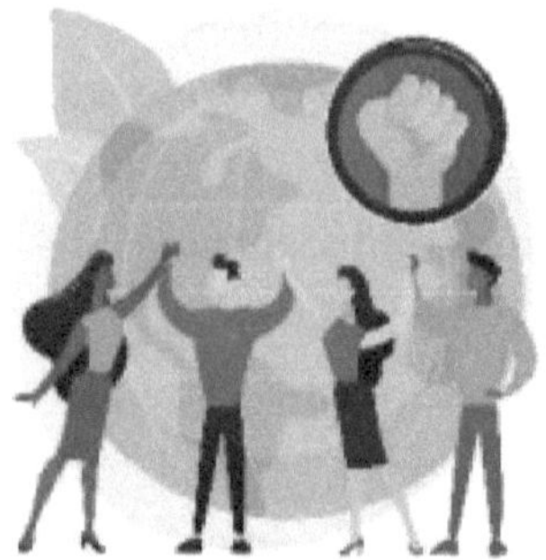

Empowering Yourself in Every Chapter of Life As we conclude this detailed exploration of living with low vision, remember that every chapter of life is an opportunity for empowerment. By integrating practical strategies, fostering emotional resilience, and leveraging supportive networks, you can navigate the journey of low vision with grace and confidence. This chapter serves as your roadmap, filled with detailed insights and friendly advice to illuminate your path. In the upcoming chapters, we'll delve deeper into advocacy, technology, and the inspiring stories of individuals who have embraced life with low vision. Embrace this chapter as a companion, a resource, and a source of inspiration on your journey of thriving with low vision.

Chapter 8: Beyond the Blurriness: Innovations in Macular Degeneration Research

Welcome to a chapter that ventures into the exciting realm of macular degeneration research—a journey where groundbreaking discoveries and innovative technologies strive to unveil the mysteries of the macula. In this detailed exploration, we will navigate the current research landscape, shedding light on promising avenues that offer hope for the future. So, let's embark on this journey together, delving into the intricate world of scientific advancements with enthusiasm and optimism.

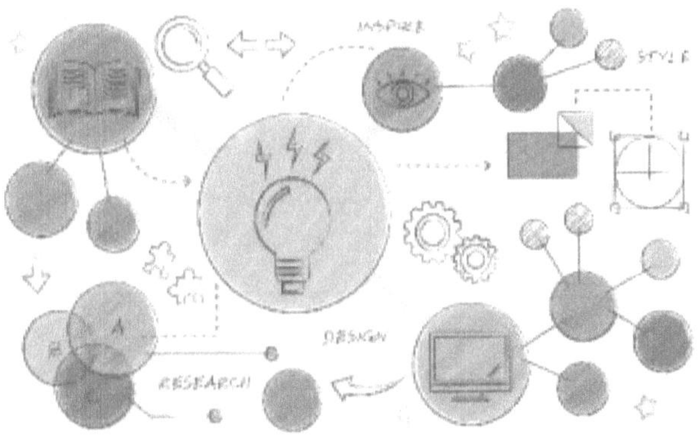

Understanding the Quest: Unraveling Macular Degeneration

The quest for understanding macular degeneration resembles a captivating puzzle, with researchers tirelessly working to decipher its complexities. This section serves as an introduction, highlighting the significance of research in unraveling the mechanisms, causes, and potential treatments for this prevalent eye condition.

1. Genetic Discoveries: Cracking the Code

Imagine genetic research as a key that unlocks the secrets encoded in our DNA. Recent advancements in genetics have revealed specific genetic variants associated with an increased risk of macular degeneration. Researchers are delving into the intricate dance of genes, striving to identify key players and understand how they contribute to the development and progression of AMD.

Understanding the genetic landscape enhances our knowledge of individual susceptibility. It paves the way for personalized treatments tailored to a person's genetic profile.

1. Stem Cell Therapy: Nurturing Hope

Stem cell therapy arises as a source of hope in the landscape of macular degeneration research. The concept involves using stem cells to replace damaged or degenerated cells in the retina, including those in the macula. Scientists are investigating the capabilities of stem cells to restore vision and slow the progression of AMD.

Though stem cell therapy is still in its initial phases of development, its promise is monumental. It represents a paradigm shift in treating macular degeneration, aiming not just to manage the condition but to rejuvenate and regenerate the damaged tissues.

Innovations in Treatment: Precision and Personalization

This section delves into innovations that aim to revolutionize the treatment landscape for macular degeneration. From cutting-edge medications to novel delivery methods, researchers are exploring avenues that prioritize precision and personalization.

1. Gene Therapy: Correcting the Blueprint

Gene therapy stands at the forefront of precision medicine, offering a targeted approach to address the underlying genetic factors contributing to macular degeneration. Researchers are developing techniques to deliver therapeutic genes into the retina, correcting or modifying genetic anomalies associated with AMD.

The potential of gene therapy lies not only in halting disease progression but also in restoring the normal functioning of the macula. As research advances, gene therapy promises to become a transformative intervention for individuals with specific genetic variants linked to AMD.

1. Drug Delivery Innovations: Beyond the Needle

Imagine a future where treatments for macular degeneration are not only practical but also less invasive. Drug delivery innovations are exploring alternatives to frequent injections, such as sustained-release implants and drug-eluting devices. These advancements aim to enhance treatment adherence and reduce the burden on individuals undergoing regular injections.

Developing sustained-release technologies opens avenues for more comfortable and convenient treatment options. It represents a significant step in making macular degeneration management more patient-friendly and accessible.

Artificial Intelligence: A Visionary Ally

Artificial intelligence (AI) emerges as a visionary ally in macular degeneration research. This section explores how AI revolutionizes AMD diagnosis, monitoring, and treatment planning.

1. AI in Diagnostics: Decoding Images with Precision

AI algorithms are trained to analyze retinal images with unprecedented precision. This capability allows for early detection of subtle changes associated with macular degeneration, enabling timely intervention. AI-powered diagnostics serve as a valuable tool for eye care professionals, enhancing their ability to identify and monitor the progression of AMD.

1. Personalized Treatment Plans: AI as a Guide

Integrating AI into personalized medicine is transforming the landscape of treatment planning. AI algorithms analyze vast datasets, including genetic information and clinical profiles, to tailor treatment plans based on individual characteristics. This approach ensures that interventions are effective and aligned with each person's unique needs and response to treatment.

Patient-Centric Research: Shaping the Future Together

In this section, we explore the growing emphasis on patient-centric research—the idea that individuals living with macular degeneration actively contribute to the research process. From participating in clinical trials to sharing valuable insights, patients play a pivotal role in shaping the future of AMD research.

1. Patient Advocacy and Engagement: A Collective Voice

Patient advocacy groups and engaged individuals are catalysts for change in macular degeneration research. Their collective voice influences research priorities, accelerates awareness, and fosters collaboration between researchers, healthcare professionals, and those directly impacted by AMD.

1. Participatory Research: Bridging the Gap

Participatory research models involve individuals with AMD in the research process. From providing input on study designs to sharing lived experiences, participants become partners in the quest for solutions. This collaborative approach ensures that research aligns with the practical needs and concerns of those it seeks to benefit.

Looking Ahead: A Future Brightened by Knowledge

As we conclude this detailed exploration of innovations in macular degeneration research, envision a future brightened by knowledge, discovery, and transformative treatments. Each breakthrough, whether in genetics, stem cell therapy, AI applications, or patient engagement, contributes to a mosaic of hope for individuals living with AMD.

This chapter is a testament to the remarkable progress in macular degeneration research and the unwavering commitment of researchers, healthcare professionals, and individuals affected by AMD. In the upcoming chapters, we'll explore lifestyle considerations, patient advocacy, and the holistic approach to managing macular degeneration. Embrace this chapter as a source of inspiration as we look forward to a future where the shadows of macular degeneration are progressively illuminated by scientific innovation.

Chapter 9: Coping with Change: Emotional and Psychological Aspects of AMD

Welcome to a chapter that delves into the emotional and psychological landscape of living with age-related macular degeneration (AMD). Coping with change, especially involving your vision, can be a multifaceted journey. In this detailed exploration, we will navigate the various aspects of emotional well-being, providing insights, coping strategies, and a friendly guide to help you navigate the emotional terrain of AMD with resilience and grace.

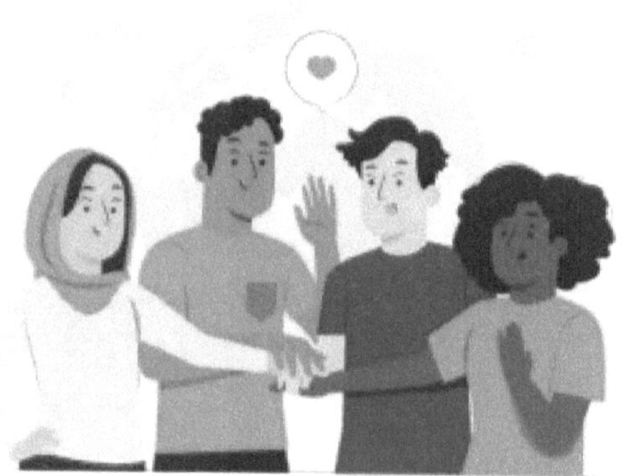

Understanding Emotional Impact: The Heart of the Matter

The emotional impact of AMD extends beyond the physical changes. This section is a compassionate exploration of the feelings and adjustments often accompanying a macular degeneration diagnosis. Recognizing the emotional nuances is the first step toward building a foundation of support.

1. Grief and Loss: Navigating a New Landscape

A diagnosis of AMD can evoke a sense of grief and loss, not only for the vision you may be losing but also for the adjustments required in various aspects of life. Acknowledging these feelings and recognizing that grieving is a natural part of adapting to change is essential.

2. Emotional Rollercoaster: Understanding the Swings

Living with AMD often involves navigating an emotional rollercoaster. Some days may bring a sense of acceptance and resilience, while others may be filled with frustration or sadness. Understanding the variability of emotions is crucial, and it's okay to embrace the highs and lows as part of the journey.

Building Emotional Resilience: A Personal Toolkit

This section explores practical strategies and tools to cultivate emotional resilience. From coping mechanisms to seeking support, these insights aim to empower you with the emotional toolkit needed to navigate the challenges AMD poses.

1. Open Communication: Sharing Your Journey

Open communication serves as a cornerstone for emotional well-being. Express your emotions to confidant friends or family, or seek support from a mental health professional. Expressing your feelings fosters understanding and creates a support network that can serve as a wellspring of strength.

1. Support Groups: Connecting with Peers

Joining a support group in person or online provides a space to connect with individuals who share similar experiences. Hearing others' stories, sharing your own, and exchanging coping strategies can be immensely valuable. Support groups cultivate a sense of community and diminish the passion for insulation.

1. Professional Counseling: A Guiding Light

Professional counseling offers a guided journey through the emotional aspects of AMD. A mental health professional experienced in supporting individuals with vision loss can provide coping strategies, emotional support, and a safe space to explore the impact of AMD on your life.

Adapting to Lifestyle Changes: A Holistic Approach

This section delves into the practical aspects of adapting to lifestyle changes prompted by AMD. From daily routines to maintaining independence, these insights aim to empower you to navigate the adjustments with a holistic perspective.

1. Assistive Technologies: Enabling Independence

Explore the world of assistive technologies designed to enhance independence. From magnifiers and audiobooks to voice-activated devices, these tools can make daily tasks more accessible. Embracing assistive technologies is not a sign of dependence but a pathway to continued autonomy.

1. Adaptive Strategies: Navigating Daily Life

Adaptive strategies involve finding alternative approaches to everyday activities. This might include adjusting lighting conditions, organizing living spaces for better navigation, or utilizing contrasting colors to enhance visibility. Minor adjustments can yield a substantial influence on maintaining a sense of normalcy.

Embracing Positive Perspectives: A Mindset of Possibilities

This section explores the power of positive thinking and cultivating a mindset that focuses on possibilities rather than limitations. From gratitude practices to reframing challenges, these perspectives aim to shift the narrative toward empowerment.

1. Gratitude Journaling: Counting Blessings

Gratitude journaling involves regularly noting down things you are thankful for. It can be a simple yet powerful practice that shifts the focus from challenges to the positive aspects of life. Cultivating gratitude can contribute to an overall sense of well-being.

1. Reframing Challenges: Shaping Perspectives

Reframing challenges involves looking at difficulties through a different lens. Instead of viewing AMD as a limitation, consider it an opportunity for personal growth, adaptability, and resilience. Shaping perspectives empowers you to find meaning and purpose despite the changes.

Navigating Relationships: Building Bridges of Understanding

This section explores the dynamics of relationships and offers insights into building bridges of understanding with family, friends, and colleagues. Effective communication and mutual support are pivotal in fostering a sense of connection amidst the changes brought about by AMD.

1. Family Dynamics: Communicating Openly

Family dynamics play a crucial role in the emotional landscape of AMD. Open communication is critical. Share your experiences, educate your loved ones about AMD, and express your needs. Building a foundation of understanding contributes to a supportive family environment.

1. Friendships and Social Life: Sustaining Connections

Social connections are vital for emotional well-being. While AMD might bring changes to social activities, finding alternative ways to engage with friends and participate in social events ensures that your support network remains robust. Sustaining connections contributes to a sense of belonging.

Looking Ahead: A Journey of Continual Adaptation

As we conclude this detailed exploration of AMD's emotional and psychological aspects, envision a continual adaptation and growth journey. Embracing change involves coping with challenges, cultivating resilience, seeking support, and maintaining a positive outlook.

This chapter serves as a companion, offering detailed insights and friendly advice to navigate the emotional landscape of AMD. In the upcoming chapters, we'll further explore lifestyle considerations, advocacy, and the ever-evolving landscape of macular degeneration research. Embrace this chapter as a source of empowerment, recognizing that the journey ahead is a canvas you paint with strength, resilience, and an unwavering belief in the possibilities beyond the blurriness.

Chapter 10: Diet and Lifestyle: A Prescription for Macular Health

Welcome to a chapter that unveils the transformative power of diet and lifestyle in nurturing the health of your precious macula. As we embark on this journey, envision these choices not merely as daily routines but as a personalized prescription that promotes resilience, vitality, and the well-being of your vision. In this detailed exploration, we will navigate the intricate connections between nutrition, lifestyle, and macular health. We will offer insights, practical tips, and a friendly guide to empower you to achieve optimal visual wellness.

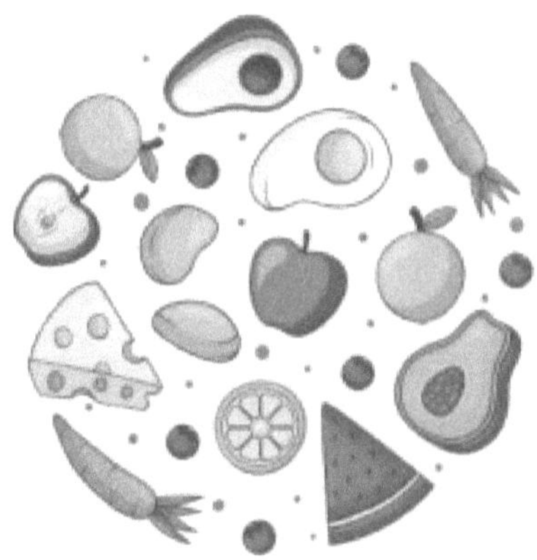

Understanding the Macula: A Marvel of Precision

Before we delve into the intricacies of diet and lifestyle, let's take a moment to appreciate the marvel that is your macula. This tiny region at the center of your retina is responsible for sharp, detailed vision. This visual masterpiece enables you to appreciate the world's beauty.

1. The Macula's Nutritional Cravings: A Balanced Symphony

Imagine the macula as a connoisseur of nutrients, craving a balanced symphony of vitamins, minerals, and antioxidants to sustain its intricate structure and functionality. This section explores the nutrients essential for macular health and their role in preserving your vision.

Your macula thrives on a palette of visionary nutrients, each contributing to its vitality. Among these, lutein and zeaxanthin, which act as the golden hues, are found abundantly in leafy greens like spinach and kale. Omega-3 fatty acids, the azure tones, are sourced from fatty fish like salmon and flaxseeds. The crimson shades, indicative of the antioxidant-rich Vitamins C and E, are present in citrus fruits, nuts, and seeds.

Crafting a Macula-Friendly Diet: The Culinary Canvas

This section transforms the principles of macular nutrition into a culinary canvas, where the art of crafting a macula-friendly diet becomes an enjoyable and flavorful experience. From vibrant salads to omega-3-rich delights, let's explore the diverse and delicious world of macula-conscious eating.

1. Leafy Greens: The Green Foundation

Leafy greens, reminiscent of the lush brushstrokes on our culinary canvas, take center stage. Spinach, kale, and collard greens abound in lutein and zeaxanthin, essential pigments that safeguard the macula from harmful ultraviolet (UV) light. Incorporate these greens into salads, smoothies, or delightful sides.

1. Fatty Fish: Oceanic Omega-3 Elegance

Imagine the oceanic elegance of fatty fish—salmon, mackerel, and trout—as bold strokes infusing your diet with omega-3 fatty acids. These fats play a role in maintaining the structural integrity of the retina, promoting optimal macular health. Grill, bake or enjoy them in savory stews for a delectable, vision-enhancing experience.

1. Colorful Fruits and Nuts: A Nutrient-Rich Mosaic

Craft a nutrient-rich mosaic with the vibrant hues of fruits and nuts. Citrus fruits, berries, and nuts provide a rich tapestry of vitamins C and E and antioxidants that combat oxidative stress. Snack on a handful of nuts or savor a fruit salad to infuse your diet with these macula-loving nutrients.

1. Whole Grains: The Foundation of Vitality

Whole grains form the foundation of vitality in our culinary canvas. Brown rice, quinoa, and total wheat products offer a spectrum of nutrients, including zinc, contributing to the macula's health. Elevate your meals with these wholesome grains, providing sustained energy and essential minerals.

Hydration and Macular Wellness: Nourishing the Oasis

In this section, we explore the role of hydration in macular wellness—a vital aspect often overlooked in the quest for optimal vision. Hydration serves as the oasis that nourishes your eyes and supports the overall health of the visual system.

1. Water: The Clear Elixir

Water, the clear elixir of life, is fundamental to maintaining macular health. Staying adequately hydrated supports the circulation of nutrients to the eyes, ensuring the macula receives its essential nourishment. Make a habit of sipping water throughout the day and infusing it with a citrus splash for added antioxidant benefits.

1. Herbal Teas: Infusions of Antioxidant Serenity

Herbal teas, with their aromatic infusions, offer a serene journey into antioxidant-rich hydration. Chamomile, green tea, and rooibos tea provide a delightful experience and antioxidants that contribute to the overall well-being of your eyes. Explore the world of herbal teas to find your favorite blends.

Lifestyle Choices and Visual Wellness: The Dance of Harmony

Beyond nutrition, lifestyle choices play a significant role in the dance of harmony that supports visual wellness. This section explores the interplay between daily habits, physical activity, and ocular health, providing insights into how lifestyle choices can influence the longevity of your vision.

1. Healthy Weight: Balancing the Equation

Maintaining a healthy weight is akin to balancing the equation of visual wellness. Excess body weight, particularly around the waist, is linked to a higher risk of macular degeneration. Cultivate a lifestyle that includes a well-balanced diet and consistent physical activity to attain and maintain a healthy weight.

1. Regular Exercise: The Rhythmic Stride

Visual wellness thrives on the rhythmic stride of regular exercise. Participate in activities that raise your heart rate and foster cardiovascular health. Whether it's brisk walking, cycling, or dancing, incorporating regular exercise into your routine enhances blood flow to the eyes, supporting macular health.

1. Eye-Friendly Habits: Blink, Rest, and Protect

Cultivate eye-friendly habits that contribute to the overall well-being of your vision. Practice the 20-20-20 rule—every 20 minutes, look at something 20 feet away for at least 20 seconds—to alleviate eye strain. Ensure your workspace is well-lit, and consider protective eyewear, especially in environments with potential hazards.

Sun Protection for Visual Radiance: Shades of Care

This section explores the importance of sun protection for visual radiance. The eyes, especially the sensitive macula, are susceptible to damage from ultraviolet (UV) rays. Embracing shades of care involves adopting practices that shield your eyes from the sun's harmful effects.

1. Sunglasses: Stylish Shields

Sunglasses are not just stylish accessories; they are shields that protect your eyes from harmful UV rays. Select sunglasses that provide 100% UVA and UVB ray protection and wear them consistently outdoors. The right shades not only enhance your visual comfort but also contribute to the long-term health of your eyes.

1. Hats and Visors: Nature's Umbrellas

Hats and visors act as nature's umbrellas, providing additional eye protection. Opt for wide-brimmed hats that cast a shadow over your face, reducing the amount of direct sunlight reaching your eyes. This simple accessory complements your sunglasses by creating a comprehensive shield against UV rays.

Sleep, Stress, and Vision: The Trifecta of Well-Being

This section explores the interconnectedness of sleep, stress, and vision. This trifecta influences your overall well-being, including the health of your eyes. Understanding their interplay and adopting practices that promote balance contribute to the longevity of your visual wellness.

1. Quality Sleep: Restorative Repose

Quality sleep is the foundation of restorative repose for your eyes. Strive for 7-9 hours of uninterrupted sleep to support the regenerative processes crucial for ocular health. Create a sleep-friendly environment, dimming lights, and minimize screen time before bedtime to enhance the quality of your rest.

1. Stress Management: Serenity Amidst Challenges

Stress management is the key to maintaining serenity amidst life's challenges. Chronic stress can contribute to eye strain and exacerbate conditions like dry eyes. Integrate stress-relief practices into your routine, such as meditation, deep breathing exercises, or hobbies that bring joy and relaxation.

Regular Eye Checkups: The Visionary Check-In

In this section, we emphasize the importance of regular eye checkups. This visionary check-in ensures proactive monitoring of your eye health. Eye exams conducted by an eye care professional play a pivotal role in detecting and managing conditions that may affect the macula. 1. Comprehensive Eye Exams: Beyond 20/20 Vision

Comprehensive eye exams extend beyond assessing 20/20 vision.

Comprehensive evaluations include a detailed assessment of your visual acuity, eye pressure, and the overall well-being of your eyes. Regular eye checkups enable early detection of potential issues, allowing timely intervention to preserve your vision.

2. Communicate Changes: Your Vision, Your Voice

Your vision is unique, and you are your best advocate. If you notice any changes in your vision or experience discomfort, communicate these changes to your eye care professional. Open and honest communication ensures that your eye care plan is tailored to your needs, promoting optimal macular health.

Holistic Approaches to Visual Wellness: A Wholesome Perspective

As we conclude this detailed exploration of diet and lifestyle for macular health, envision a wholesome perspective that embraces the interconnectedness of nutrition, lifestyle choices, and holistic well-being. Each choice you make—from the foods on your plate to the habits you cultivate—contributes to the vitality of your macula and the longevity of your visual wellness.

This chapter serves as a friendly guide, offering information and an invitation to embark on a journey of personalized care for your eyes. In the upcoming chapters, we'll further explore lifestyle considerations, advocacy, and the ever-evolving landscape of macular degeneration research. Embrace this chapter as your prescription for macular health, recognizing that every choice you make is a brushstroke on the canvas of your visual well-being—a masterpiece you create with care, intention, and an unwavering belief in the radiant possibilities ahead.

Chapter 11: Sight-Saving Technologies: Tools for Independence

Welcome to a chapter that unveils the marvels of sight-saving technologies—innovations designed to empower and enhance the independence of individuals facing the challenges of visual impairment. In this detailed exploration, we will navigate through a world of cutting-edge tools and assistive devices, each crafted to open new avenues of accessibility, autonomy, and possibility. So, let's embark on a journey where technology becomes a beacon of hope, a guide to independence, and a companion on the path to a life without limits.

The Transformative Power of Assistive Technologies: A Prelude

Before we dive into the specifics, let's take a moment to appreciate the transformative power of assistive technologies. These tools are not merely gadgets but gateways to a world where barriers dissolve, and possibilities unfold. From enhancing daily activities to fostering connectivity, assistive technologies are the threads that weave a tapestry of independence.

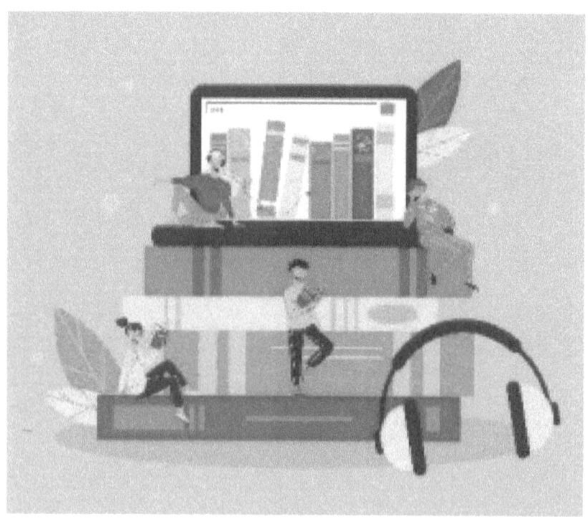

1. The Digital Revolution: A Visionary Landscape

In the era of the digital revolution, technology serves as a visionary landscape, offering a multitude of tools tailored to address the unique needs of individuals with visual impairment. This section explores the diverse categories of assistive technologies that have emerged, from those designed for everyday tasks to those fostering a seamless digital experience.

Navigating the Everyday: Tools for Daily Independence

This section delves into tools that enhance daily activities, making them more accessible and enjoyable. From reading to cooking, these technologies are designed to integrate seamlessly into your routine, empowering you to navigate the everyday confidently.

1. Talking Book Libraries: A Symphony of Narratives

Enter the world of talking book libraries, where literature comes alive through the power of narration. Audiobooks and podcasts provide a symphony of narratives, allowing you to indulge in the joy of literature without the constraints of traditional print. Whether you're into action or non-action or exploring the latest bestsellers, talking book libraries are your gateway to a world of literary exploration.

1. Smart Home Assistants: Your Digital Concierge

Imagine a home where your every command is met with instant, intuitive responses. Smart home assistants, like Amazon's Alexa and Google Assistant, serve as your digital concierge, helping you control lights, set reminders, and even read the news through voice commands. Embrace the convenience of a connected home that adapts to your needs.

1. Braille Displays: Feel the Words Come Alive

For those who cherish the tactile beauty of language, braille displays offer a way to feel the words come alive. These devices connect to your digital devices, converting on-screen text into braille and allowing you to read emails, documents, and more with your fingertips. Braille displays bridge the gap between traditional literacy and the digital age.

Digital Inclusion: Connectivity in the Palm of Your Hand

As technology continues to evolve, digital inclusion becomes a cornerstone of independence. This section explores tools that foster connectivity, ensuring that you remain seamlessly integrated into the digital landscape, whether it's through social interactions, navigation, or staying informed.

1. Accessible Smartphones: Your Pocket-Sized Hub

Smartphones have become more than communication devices; they are pocket-sized hubs of accessibility. Accessible features, such as screen readers, voice assistants, and magnification options, transform smartphones into assertive communication, navigation, and information retrieval tools. Your smartphone becomes a window to the world, connecting you to many possibilities.

1. Voice Recognition Software: Turning Words into Actions

With remarkable accuracy, voice recognition software turns spoken words into decisive actions. Whether you're drafting emails, composing documents, or commanding your device, the power of your voice becomes a catalyst for productivity. Embrace the freedom of hands-free interaction and let your words shape the digital landscape around you.

1. Navigation Apps: Charting Paths with Precision

Navigate the world confidently using specialized navigation apps designed for individuals with visual impairment. These apps provide detailed auditory instructions, real-time location information, and even detect nearby points of interest. From exploring new neighborhoods to independently navigating public transportation, these apps put the power of precise navigation in the palm of your hand.

Visual Magnification and Enhancement: Seeing the Details

For those moments when visual magnification and enhancement are essential, a range of technologies stands ready to assist. This section explores tools that amplify the details, allowing you to see and engage with the world around you with clarity and precision.

1. Electronic Magnifiers: Zooming into Clarity

Electronic magnifiers, also known as video magnifiers, bring the power of zoom into your hands. These handheld devices or desktop solutions magnify text, images, and objects, providing a clear and detailed view. Whether reading a menu or examining a photo, electronic magnifiers amplify the details and clarify your visual experience.

1. OCR Apps: Reading the Unseen

Optical Character Recognition (OCR) apps transform printed text into spoken words, making the unseen accessible. Point your smartphone's camera at a document, and the app will read the text aloud. From restaurant menus to product labels, OCR apps empower you to access printed information independently in various contexts.

Beyond Vision: Tools for Environmental Awareness

This section explores technologies that extend beyond traditional visual enhancement, focusing on tools that enhance your environmental awareness. From detecting obstacles to recognizing faces, these innovations provide an extra layer of information, fostering a heightened sense of autonomy in various settings.

1. Wearable Devices: A Sixth Sense

Wearable devices, equipped with sensors and cameras, act as a sixth sense, providing real-time information about your surroundings. From identifying faces to warning about obstacles, these devices enhance your spatial awareness, offering additional information as you move through the world. Whether a pair of smart glasses or a wearable clip-on device, these innovations empower you to navigate your environment confidently.

1. Object Recognition Apps: Identifying the Unseen

Object recognition apps leverage the power of artificial intelligence to identify and describe objects in your environment. Point your smartphone's camera at an object; the app will provide auditory feedback about what it sees. From distinguishing between cans in your pantry to identifying colors, object recognition apps bring a new level of independence to daily life.

Embracing the Future: Innovations on the Horizon

As we conclude this exploration of sight-saving technologies, let's glance toward the future—where innovation knows no bounds. Emerging technologies, from advanced wearables to cutting-edge artificial intelligence, promise to revolutionize the accessibility landscape further. The future holds the potential for even more sophisticated tools that empower individuals with visual impairment to lead lives of unparalleled independence.

This chapter isn't just a companion to assistive technologies; it's an assignment to embrace a world where invention becomes a lamp of stopgap, a ground to independence, and a testament to the bottomless capabilities of the mortal spirit. In the forthcoming chapters, we'll further explore diurnal living, advocacy, and the evolving geography of macular degeneration exploration. So, let technology be your supporter on this trip — a companion that opens doors, breaks walls, and titleholders your right to a life without limits.

Chapter 12: Support Systems: Building a Network for Those with Macular Degeneration

Welcome to a chapter that illuminates the importance of support systems in the journey of individuals facing macular degeneration. In the vast tapestry of managing this condition, having a robust support network is not just valuable; it's a lifeline. This detailed exploration will delve into the various facets of building and nurturing a support system tailored for those navigating macular degeneration challenges. Let's embark on a journey where connection, understanding, and encouragement become the pillars of strength.

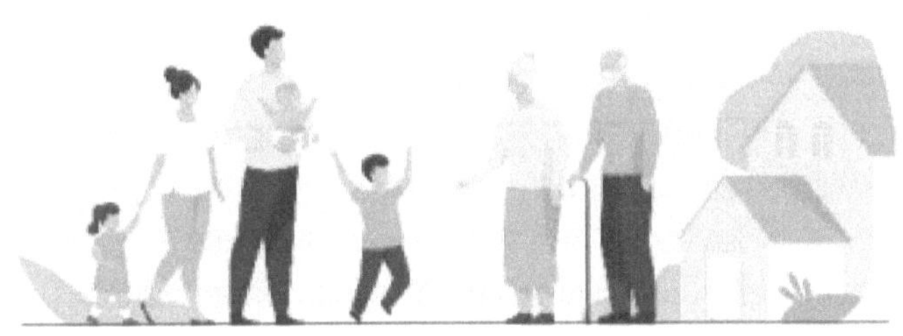

Understanding the Power of Support: A Prelude

Before we delve into the specifics, let's take a moment to recognize the profound impact a supportive network can have on those dealing with macular degeneration. It's more than just assistance; it's the essence of shared understanding, empathy, and a collective commitment to facing challenges head-on. A support system is a bedrock upon which individuals can find solace, information, and the resilience needed to thrive despite the hurdles.

1. The Role of Family: A Pillar of Unconditional Support

Family is often the first line of support, providing a foundation of unconditional love and understanding. This section explores how family members can play a pivotal role in the journey of someone with macular degeneration, offering emotional and practical support.

Emotional Support: Nurturing the Heart

Family members become emotional anchors, offering reassurance and understanding in the face of uncertainty. Whether through open conversations, shared experiences, or simply being present, the emotional support of family members establishes a secure environment where individuals feel comfortable expressing their feelings and concerns.

Practical Support: From Everyday Tasks to Adaptations

Beyond emotions, family support extends to practical aspects of daily living. From assisting with household tasks to exploring adaptive technologies and making necessary home modifications, family members become partners in creating an environment that fosters independence and accessibility.

1. Friends as Allies: The Strength of Companionship

This section delves into the significance of friendships as vital components of a robust support system. Friends, whether longstanding or newfound, contribute to the social fabric that enhances the quality of life for individuals with macular degeneration.

Understanding: Friends Who See Beyond Vision

True friends see beyond vision challenges, understanding without judgment. This section explores how genuine friendships contribute to a sense of normalcy, humor, and shared experiences that transcend the limitations posed by macular degeneration.

Inclusion: Friends in Social Activities

Friends play a crucial role in promoting social inclusion. Whether engaging in activities like book clubs, outings, or hobbies, friends become allies in creating enjoyable experiences, fostering a sense of belonging, and combating isolation.

1. Peer Support Groups: Community Connection and Shared Wisdom

This section emphasizes the significance of peer support groups—a community of individuals who share similar experiences and challenges. Peer support is a powerful force that provides empathy, shared wisdom, and a platform for individuals to learn and grow together.

Emotional Resonance: Shared Experiences and Understanding

Peer support groups create a space where individuals share their experiences, fears, and triumphs without judgment. This emotional resonance builds a sense of camaraderie, knowing that others understand the unique journey of living with macular degeneration.

Practical Guidance: Navigating Challenges Together

Beyond emotional connection, peer support groups offer practical guidance. From sharing tips on adaptive technologies to discussing coping strategies, the group's collective wisdom becomes a valuable resource for navigating the daily challenges of macular degeneration.

1. Professional Support: Collaboration with Healthcare Teams

This section highlights the importance of professional support from healthcare teams, including ophthalmologists, low-vision specialists, and rehabilitation professionals. Collaboration with these professionals is essential for comprehensive care and tailored strategies to manage macular degeneration.

Ophthalmologists: Partners in Ocular Health

Building a solid relationship with ophthalmologists is critical to managing macular degeneration effectively. Regular check-ups, open communication, and a collaborative approach ensure that individuals receive timely interventions and personalized care plans.

Low Vision Specialists: Navigating Visual Challenges

Low vision specialists play a crucial role in enhancing visual function and independence. Through assessments, customized visual aids, and training, they empower individuals to adapt to changes in vision, maximizing their ability to perform daily tasks.

Rehabilitation Professionals: Skill-Building for Independence

Rehabilitation professionals, including orientation and mobility specialists, occupational therapists, and counselors, contribute to skill-building for independence. Whether learning mobility techniques, adapting workspaces, or addressing emotional well-being, these professionals offer holistic support.

1. Online Communities: The Digital Thread of Connection

In this digital age, online communities are integral to support systems. This section explores the benefits of connecting with others through online forums, social media groups, and virtual platforms, fostering a sense of global community.

Shared Knowledge: Tapping into Global Insights

Online communities grant access to a treasure trove of shared knowledge. Individuals can tap into global insights, learn about the latest advancements, and discover practical tips from a diverse community of people navigating similar challenges.

Emotional Encouragement: Virtual Shoulder to Lean On

The digital thread of connection extends beyond knowledge-sharing to emotional encouragement. Online communities grow a virtual shoulder to lean on, creating a space where individuals can express their thoughts and seek advice and understanding from those who have walked a similar path.

1. Advocacy Groups: Amplifying Voices for Change

This section emphasizes the role of advocacy groups in amplifying the voices of those affected by macular degeneration. Individuals can raise awareness, drive research, and influence policies that benefit the macular degeneration community by participating in advocacy efforts.

Awareness Campaigns: Shaping Public Perception

Advocacy groups are essential in shaping public perception through awareness campaigns. Individuals can change the narrative around macular degeneration by sharing personal stories, disseminating information, and engaging with the media.

Research Initiatives: Driving Innovation and Progress

Active participation in advocacy groups supports research initiatives. By joining forces with researchers, individuals can drive innovation, fund studies, and accelerate progress toward discovering improved treatments and, ultimately, a cure for macular degeneration.

Conclusion: The Tapestry of Support

As we conclude this detailed exploration of support systems for those with macular degeneration, envision a tapestry woven with threads of connection, understanding, and encouragement. Building and nurturing a robust support system is not a solitary journey; it's a collective effort that enriches the lives of individuals facing macular degeneration and those who stand beside them. Each support element—whether from family, friends, peers, professionals, online communities, or advocacy groups—contributes to a resilient network that empowers individuals to live whole and meaningful lives despite the challenges. Embrace the strength that comes from connection, for in unity, there is a richness that transcends the limitations posed by macular degeneration. In the upcoming chapters, we'll further explore aspects of daily living, innovative technologies, and the evolving landscape of macular degeneration research. Let this chapter be a testament to the transformative power of support. This force illuminates the path toward a life filled with possibility and connection.

Chapter 13: Advocacy and Awareness: Shining a Light on Macular Degeneration

Welcome to a chapter dedicated to the power of advocacy and awareness in macular degeneration. In this exploration, we will delve into advocacy's crucial role in driving change, shaping policies, influencing change, and amplifying the voices of those affected by this condition. Additionally, we'll highlight the significance of awareness campaigns in reshaping public perception, fostering understanding, and ultimately paving the way toward a future without macular degeneration. Come with us on this journey as we illuminate the path to advocacy, one that is grounded in compassion, resilience, and a shared commitment to a world free from the constraints of macular degeneration.

Understanding the Essence of Advocacy: A Prelude

Before we dive into the specifics, let's examine the essence of advocacy and its profound impact on the landscape of macular degeneration. Advocacy is more than a call for change; it is a collective voice that seeks to challenge perceptions, break down barriers, and drive progress. It is the catalyst for transformation, rooted in the belief that every individual affected by macular degeneration deserves a future filled with possibilities. This chapter unfolds the tapestry of advocacy, weaving together stories of resilience, initiatives for change, and the unwavering dedication of those who champion the cause.

1. The Power of Personal Stories: Advocacy Starts with You

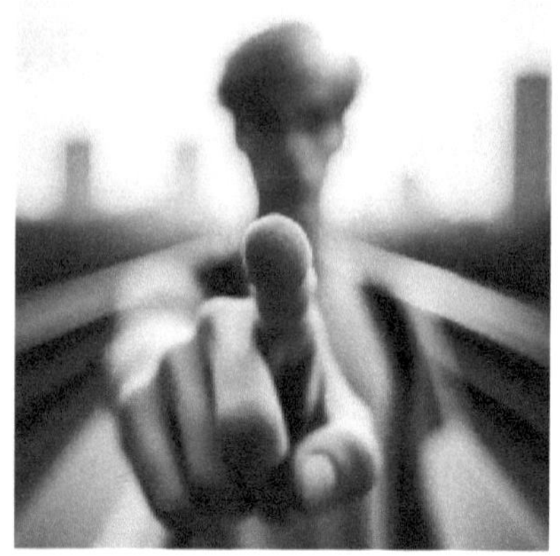

This section emphasizes the extraordinary influence of personal stories in advocacy efforts. Whether you are someone directly affected by macular degeneration or a caregiver, sharing your story becomes a powerful tool for raising awareness, fostering empathy, and inspiring action.

Sharing Journeys: The Human Face of Macular Degeneration

Your journey is waiting to be told—a story that resonates with others facing similar challenges. By sharing your experiences, you humanize the impact of macular degeneration, making it relatable and compelling for a broader audience.

Building Empathy: Creating Connections through Narratives

Personal stories have the unique ability to build empathy. They transcend statistics and medical terms, creating connections between individuals and those unfamiliar with the nuances of macular degeneration. Your narrative becomes a bridge that fosters understanding and compassion.

1. Grassroots Advocacy: Mobilizing Communities for Change

This section explores the grassroots movements and community-based initiatives that form the backbone of advocacy. From local support groups to community events, grassroots advocacy empowers individuals to create change on a small scale, collectively contributing to a larger impact.

Community Support Groups: Strength in Unity

Local support groups become hubs of grassroots advocacy, offering a platform for individuals to share resources, information, and experiences. Through collective action, these groups become catalysts for change within their communities.

Community Events: Engaging the Public

Organizing and participating in community events is a dynamic way to engage the public. From informational sessions to awareness walks, these events disseminate crucial information and create spaces for dialogue and collaboration.

1. Digital Advocacy: Harnessing the Power of Online Platforms

In this digital age, online platforms play a pivotal role in advocacy. This section delves into the impact of social media, blogs, and other digital channels in amplifying the voices of individuals affected by macular degeneration and fostering a global community of advocates.

Social Media Campaigns: A Global Amplifier

Social media platforms serve as global amplifiers for advocacy efforts. Campaigns, hashtags, and shared content reach diverse audiences, creating a ripple effect that disseminates awareness, inspires engagement, and sparks conversations.

Online Communities: Uniting Advocates Worldwide

Online spaces such as forums and social media groups become virtual hubs where advocates worldwide connect. These communities provide a support network, share information, and collectively advocate for change on a broader scale.

1. Collaborative Advocacy: Partnering with Organizations and

Professionals

Collaboration is at the heart of impactful advocacy. This section explores how individuals can collaborate with organizations, healthcare professionals, and researchers to amplify their efforts and drive meaningful change.

Partnerships with Healthcare Professionals: Bridging Gaps in Knowledge

Building partnerships with healthcare professionals bridges advocacy and the medical community. By fostering collaboration, advocates contribute to a shared pool of knowledge, ensuring that medical practices align with the evolving needs of individuals with macular degeneration.

Engaging with Research Organizations: Driving Innovation

Advocates can be crucial in driving innovation by collaborating with research organizations. Supporting and participating in research initiatives contribute to developing breakthrough treatments and, ultimately, finding a cure for macular degeneration.

1. Advocacy in Legislation: Influencing Policies for Change

This section underscores the impact of advocacy in shaping policies that directly impact individuals with macular degeneration. Advocates can engage with lawmakers, join advocacy organizations, and participate in legislative initiatives to drive systemic change.

Lobbying for Change: A Voice in Legislative Halls

Advocacy extends into legislative halls, where individuals can lobby for policies that cater to the needs of those with macular degeneration. By engaging with lawmakers, advocates contribute to developing laws that enhance accessibility, healthcare, and support systems.

Joining Advocacy Organizations: Strength in Numbers

Advocacy organizations play a pivotal role in consolidating efforts and leveraging the collective strength of advocates. Joining these organizations provides individuals with a structured platform to contribute to advocacy initiatives, access resources, and participate in strategic campaigns.

1. Awareness Campaigns: Illuminating the Path to Understanding

This section focuses on the role of awareness campaigns in reshaping public perception, dispelling myths, and fostering a culture of understanding around macular degeneration. By leveraging various mediums, advocates can shine a light on the condition and its impact.

Media Campaigns: Captivating Audiences

Engaging with traditional and digital media is a powerful strategy in awareness campaigns. Advertisements, articles, and interviews can captivate audiences, educating them about macular degeneration and encouraging empathy and support.

Creative Initiatives: Art, Culture, and Macular Degeneration

Creativity becomes a potent tool in awareness campaigns. Artistic initiatives, cultural events, and collaborations with creative communities bring macular degeneration into the public consciousness in unique and impactful ways.

Conclusion: Advocacy in Action

As we conclude this detailed exploration of advocacy and awareness, envision a world where the voices of individuals with macular degeneration echo across communities, legislative halls, and digital landscapes. Advocacy is not a solitary endeavor but a collective symphony of voices, each note contributing to a melody of change. In the forthcoming chapters, we will delve further into unraveling the multifaceted aspects of macular degeneration, from innovative technologies to the daily strategies for living with low vision. Let this chapter be an inspiration—an invitation to become an advocate, a storyteller, and a beacon of light in the journey toward a world where macular degeneration is understood, resources are accessible, and a cure is within reach. Together, we shine a light on macular degeneration, illuminating a path of compassion, resilience, and hope.

Chapter 14: Looking Forward: Hopeful Perspectives on Research and Treatment

Welcome to a chapter filled with optimism as we explore the exciting realms of research and treatment for macular degeneration. In this detailed journey, we will navigate the latest advancements, innovative approaches, and the promising future that awaits those affected by this condition. With a backdrop of hope, let's delve into the intricate landscape of scientific progress, groundbreaking therapies, and the collective efforts that illuminate the path toward a brighter tomorrow.

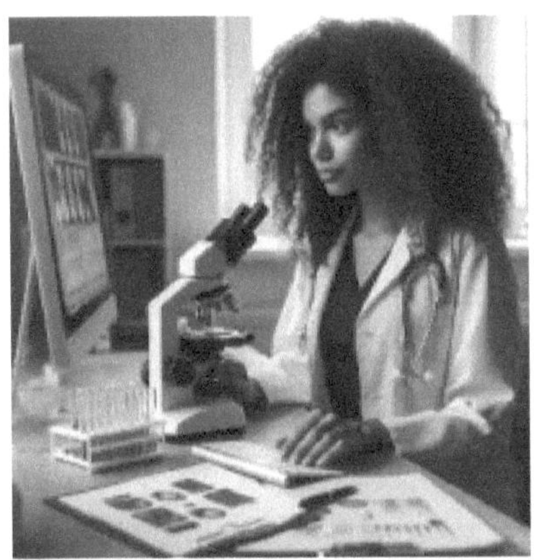

Understanding the Dynamics of Macular Degeneration Research: A Prelude

Before we explore cutting-edge research and evolving treatments, let's set the stage by understanding the dynamic nature of macular degeneration research. This chapter celebrates the tireless efforts of researchers, medical professionals, and advocates who tirelessly contribute to unraveling the mysteries of this condition. It is a testament to the collective commitment to transforming the landscape of macular degeneration from a challenge to a conquerable frontier.

1. The Evolution of Research: Tracing the Journey

This section traces the evolution of macular degeneration research, providing insights into the historical milestones that have shaped our understanding of the condition. The research journey has paved the way for contemporary breakthroughs, from discovering risk factors to developing diagnostic tools.

Discovery of Genetic Factors: Unraveling the Blueprint

Researchers have made substantial strides in comprehending the genetic factors contributing to macular degeneration. Genetic studies have unraveled crucial information about predisposition, laying the groundwork for treatments customized to individuals and preventive strategies based on an individual's genetic blueprint.

Advancements in Diagnostic Tools: Seeing Beyond the Surface

The development of advanced diagnostic tools has transformed our ability to detect macular degeneration in its early stages. From high-resolution imaging techniques to sophisticated screening technologies, these tools empower healthcare professionals to intervene proactively, potentially slowing the condition's progression.

2. Breakthrough Therapies: From Concept to Reality

This section delves into the groundbreaking therapies emerging as beacons of hope for those with macular degeneration. From pharmacological interventions to cutting-edge surgical procedures, these therapies showcase the transformative potential of modern medicine.

Anti-VEGF Treatments: Halting the Progression

Anti-VEGF (Vascular Endothelial Growth Factor) treatments have revolutionized the management of wet macular degeneration. By suppressing the abnormal growth of blood vessels, these therapies help preserve vision and, in some cases, even improve visual acuity—continual research endeavors to enhance and broaden the applications of anti-VEGF treatments.

Cell-Based Therapies: Harnessing the Power of Regeneration

Cell-based therapies, including stem cell treatments, hold immense promise in regenerating damaged retinal cells. Researchers are exploring ways to harness cells' regenerative potential to replace those affected by macular degeneration, offering a glimpse into a future where vision restoration becomes a reality.

Surgical Innovations: Precision and Restoration

Advancements in surgical techniques enhance the precision and effectiveness of interventions for macular degeneration. From retinal implants to microsurgical procedures, these innovations are on the frontier of restoring vision and improving the quality of life for individuals with advanced stages of the condition.

1. Targeted Therapies: Precision in Action

This section explores the concept of targeted therapies, where treatments are customized to the specific characteristics of an individual's macular degeneration. Precision medicine is emerging as a paradigm shift, recognizing the unique aspects of each case and tailoring interventions for maximum efficacy.

Personalized Medicine: Tailoring Treatments to Individuals

The era of personalized medicine is upon us, macular degeneration research. By understanding patients' genetic and molecular makeup, healthcare professionals can customize treatments, optimizing outcomes and minimizing side effects.

Gene Therapy: Correcting the Blueprint

Gene therapy can correct the genetic anomalies associated with macular degeneration. By precisely altering the genetic code, researchers are exploring avenues to address the root causes of the condition, opening doors to transformative treatments that target the source of the problem.

1. Vision Restoration: Beyond Preservation

This section envisions a future where the focus shifts from merely preserving vision to actively restoring it. Through neuroprotective strategies, retinal regeneration, and neuroenhancement, researchers are exploring avenues to halt degeneration and promote the restoration of visual function.

Neuroprotective Approaches: Safeguarding Retinal Health

Neuroprotective strategies aim to safeguard the health of retinal cells, slowing down degeneration and preserving vision. From antioxidants to neuroenhancing drugs, these approaches hold promise in maintaining the vitality of the macula and sustaining visual function.

Retinal Regeneration: Paving the Way for Renewal

Research into retinal regeneration seeks to stimulate the growth and replacement of damaged retinal cells. Through a combination of cell-based therapies, growth factors, and tissue engineering, scientists are delving into methods to encourage the renewal of retinal tissue and potentially restore vision.

1. Collaborative Initiatives: The Power of Global Partnerships

This section underscores the importance of collaborative initiatives in advancing macular degeneration research. International partnerships, interdisciplinary collaborations, and the involvement of diverse stakeholders are instrumental in accelerating progress and ensuring that promising discoveries reach those who need them.

International Research Consortia: Uniting Global E orts

International research consortia bring together experts worldwide, fostering collaboration and knowledge exchange. These initiatives accelerate discovery and bring us closer to effective treatments by pooling resources, sharing data, and coordinating efforts.

Patient Involvement: A Catalyst for Progress

Active involvement of patients in research is a catalyst for progress. Patient advocacy groups, clinical trial

participation and direct engagement with individuals affected by macular degeneration play pivotal roles in shaping research agendas, ensuring that studies align with the real-world needs and aspirations of those living with the condition.

1. Future Horizons: A Glimpse into Tomorrow

This section offers a glimpse into the future horizons of macular degeneration research and treatment. From artificial intelligence applications in diagnostics to emerging technologies, we explore the possibilities, painting a picture of a future where macular degeneration is manageable and conquerable.

Artificial Intelligence in Diagnostics: Precision at Its Pinnacle

Integrating artificial intelligence (AI) in diagnostics is poised to revolutionize the early detection and monitoring of macular degeneration. AI algorithms, trained on vast datasets, can analyze imaging scans with unparalleled accuracy, enabling swift and precise diagnoses that empower timely interventions.

Emerging Technologies: Shaping the Landscape

As technology evolves, emerging innovations hold promise in shaping the landscape of macular degeneration research and treatment. From smart glasses that enhance visual perception to augmented reality applications, these technologies are on the frontier of providing practical solutions for individuals with low vision.

Conclusion: Navigating Hopeful Horizons

As we conclude this detailed exploration of research and treatment for macular degeneration, envision a horizon where scientific breakthroughs and innovative therapies converge to redefine the possibilities for individuals facing this condition. The journey is one of collaboration, dedication, and the collective pursuit of a future where macular degeneration is not a barrier but a challenge that has been met with resilience and triumph.

In the upcoming chapters, we will go deeper into various aspects of living with macular degeneration, from practical strategies for daily life to the emotional dimensions of the journey. Let this chapter be a beacon of hope—a testament to the remarkable progress and the unwavering commitment of the global community to transform the landscape of macular degeneration. Together, we navigate the hopeful horizons that await, where the promise of a brighter tomorrow becomes a reality for all.

Chapter 15: Closing Thoughts: A Vision for a Brighter Future with Macular Degeneration

As we embark on the closing chapter of our journey, we pen these thoughts with heartfelt reflection and an optimistic gaze toward the future. Our exploration into the multifaceted world of macular degeneration has been a tapestry woven with knowledge, compassion, and the shared determination to navigate the challenges posed by this condition. In this chapter, we take a moment to distill the essence of our collective journey and envision a future where the shadows of macular degeneration are cast aside. The light of hope illuminates the path forward.

Reflecting on the Journey: A Tapestry of Resilience

Our journey has been a testament to the resilience of the human spirit. Through the detailed chapters exploring the anatomy of sight, the science behind macular degeneration, and the myriad strategies for coping and living vibrantly, we have witnessed the strength inherent in each individual facing this condition. The personal stories, the triumphs over challenges, and the unwavering support from communities have collectively woven a tapestry that celebrates survival and the thriving spirit that defines those living with macular degeneration.

1. A Glimpse into Progress: From Research to Real-World Impact

As we gaze toward the future, let's acknowledge the remarkable progress in understanding, diagnosing, and treating macular degeneration. The chapters dedicated to research and treatment shed light on groundbreaking therapies, innovative approaches, and the collaborative efforts that propel us toward a future where the impact of macular degeneration is minimized.

Hopeful Horizons: Emerging Technologies and Treatment Paradigms

The glimpses into emerging technologies, personalized treatments, and breakthrough therapies offer a vision of a future where individuals with macular degeneration not only manage their condition but experience a restoration of vision and a higher quality of life. The future holds promise for transformative possibilities, from artificial intelligence aiding in diagnostics to gene therapies correcting the underlying causes.

1. Advocacy as a Driving Force: Shaping Policies and Narratives

Throughout our exploration, advocacy emerged as a driving force for change. From grassroots initiatives to legislative efforts, the collective voice of advocates has been instrumental in shaping policies, fostering awareness, and creating a supportive ecosystem for those affected by macular degeneration.

Building Bridges: Collaboration and Awareness Initiatives

Continuing collaborative efforts at the local and global levels will be pivotal as we look ahead. Building bridges between advocacy groups, healthcare professionals, researchers, and individuals will amplify the impact of awareness initiatives. These collaborative endeavors are the threads that weave a fabric of understanding, compassion, and collective action.

1. Living with Macular Degeneration: Strategies for Resilience

Our exploration into daily coping strategies for macular degeneration underscored the importance of resilience, adaptability, and a supportive community. The chapters dedicated to coping mechanisms, low vision strategies, and the emotional dimensions of the journey provided practical insights and heartfelt narratives illuminating the path for those navigating similar challenges.

Empowering Lives: Personal Stories and Practical Strategies

The personal stories in the chapters on living with low vision and coping with change serve as beacons of inspiration. From practical strategies for daily life to emotional well-being, the experiences shared by individuals with macular degeneration paint a vivid picture of empowerment, resilience, and the capacity to find beauty and joy in life's journey.

1. Looking Forward: Navigating Hopeful Horizons

In our exploration of research and treatment, we ventured into the realm of possibilities—possibilities that hold the promise of a brighter tomorrow. The chapters on breakthrough therapies, personalized medicine, and collaborative research initiatives showcased the dynamism of the scientific community and the potential for transformative advancements.

The Road Ahead: A Shared Vision for Progress

As we close this chapter, let's carry forward a shared vision for progress. A vision where research continues to unveil new horizons, treatments become more targeted and effective, and the collective voice of advocacy resonates even louder. Together, we envision a future where macular degeneration is not merely managed but where individuals thrive, supported by a community that understands, cares, and works tirelessly toward a world where the warmth of hope and possibility replaces the shadows of macular degeneration.

Conclusion: A Tapestry of Hope and Unity

In closing, let this chapter reflect the tapestry we've woven—a tapestry interwoven with threads of hope, resilience, and unity. The journey with macular degeneration is not one walked alone but a shared exploration of triumphs and challenges. As we part ways, let us carry forward the lessons learned, the insights gained, and the collective commitment to a future where the world sees the challenges and the indomitable spirit of those living with macular degeneration. The road ahead is illuminated by the light of shared knowledge, compassionate understanding, and the unwavering hope for a brighter future.

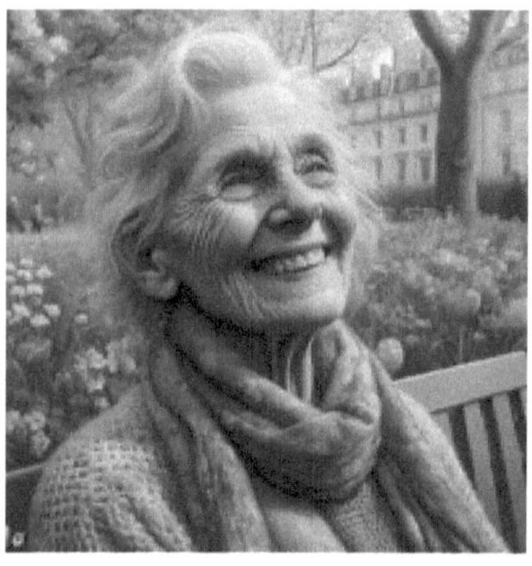

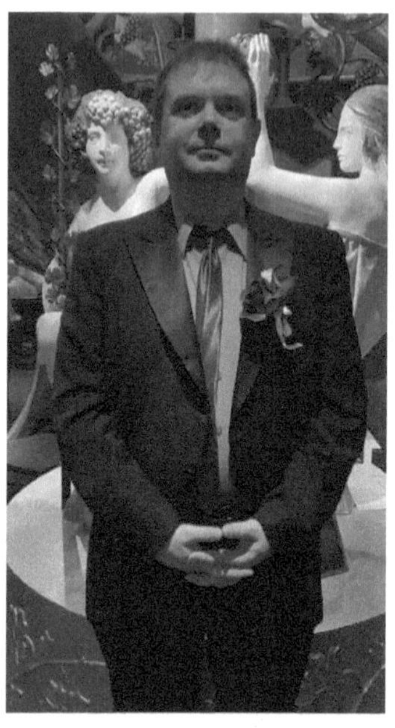

About the Author

Introducing Rodney, a passionate and versatile individual interested in various domains. He is one of the creative forces behind www.randrservices.blog, where he shares insights, expertise, and valuable information on health and wellness.

Read more at https://www.randrservices.blog/.